At the heart my fight

Mélanie Lebihain

At my heart of my fight

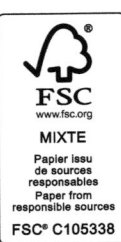

© 2020 Mélanie Lebihain

Éditeur : BoD-Books on Demand
12-14 rond-point des Champs-Élysées, 75008 Paris
Impression : Books on Demand, Norderstedt, Allemagne

Illustration : Mélanie Lebihain

ISBN : 978-2-3222-5274-9
Dépôt légal : Octobre 2020

ACKNOWLEDGEMENTS

I would like to thank the following people:

- My family and Sylvie for their unwavering support
- The stretcher bearers as well as the entire medical staff for their daily kindness
- The AR Coeur en Action Association and its Founding President for initiating this project to translate my book "Au Coeur de mon Combat".
- Léa SONZA for translating my entire book "Au Coeur de mon Combat"

CHAPTER 1. THE APPOINTMENT THAT CHANGED MY LIFE

The story I am sharing with you today is about my fight against breast cancer, a disease that affects so many women.

I am writing it to help people who are going through the same hardship, as well as to help their families and friends, who often cannot even begin to imagine what it is like. My goal is to raise awareness among the affected people, and to provide them with useful information.

I am also doing it as a method of self-expression, using what happened to me to move forward. Because it changed me. I came out of it with a renewed vitality, and a mind filled with new priorities.

Here is my story. The same story that so many women, men and even children have been through, as unfortunately, too many people are still suffering from a wide range of cancers.

It was a routine gynaecological check-up that would turn my life upside-down. On the 27th of December 2017, my gynaecologist discovered two lumps in my left breast. I had not noticed them. I had not noticed anything at all. I had however been eperiencing severe headaches quite often and had also been feeling tired. But I never would have imagined why. I used to put the blame on my work, to which I was fully committed. After a mammary ultrasound scan, I was told that the lumps were probably just benign fibroadenomae.

The radiologist even wrote down in her report the following words: 'discussion about light monitoring, full ACR3 with ultrasound scan in about four months or, more likely, follow-up with a micro-biopsy treatment subject to the gynaecologist's opinion'. Luckily for me, she decided to schedule an ultrasound scan with a specialist as quickly as possible. The scan results would say the same words: 'mammary ultrasound scan corroborating the existence of a small nodular hypo-echogenic formation indicative of a fibroadenoma, for which a puncture biopsy under the monitoring of an ultrasound scan should be scheduled'. The radiologist even told me that there was only a one percent probability for it to be cancerous. It should have reassured me. Unfortunately, my fears lingered with me right up to the day the verdict was given.

On the day of the biopsy, the radiologist, the same man who was not worried a few days prior, seemed more tensed, and a little more distant. His eye contact was brief, his answers unclear. It reinforced my intuition about the tumour being cancerous.

The results of the biopsy would be ready in about two weeks, a period with would feel much longer.

I should introduce myself. I am a thirty-two-year-old, young woman. I am married, and the mother of two children, a girl of six and a boy of three. I have been a playschool assistant for a few months now and little by little I'm discovering the pleasure of balancing my job and my personal life. Besides my son, three other toddlers keep me busy all day.

Furthermore, we are building a new house. The loan has been approved and the construction is progressing quickly. We are supposed to move into our new home next April.

I am living a very fulfilling life in my opinion: a great relationship, a loving family and a job I like. Things could not be better, and I am content.

Some words about my personality now. I am down-to-earth and hard-working. I like planning ahead. I would even say that I do not like the unknown. Not knowing what is going to happen makes me nervous. I am easily stressed-out, sometimes to an extent that makes me sick. Since my teenage years I have been trying to get rid of this part of me. A therapist helped me when I was in high school, giving me Erikstonian hypnosis sessions. The therapy was about reaching out to my subconscious in order to remove the negative thoughts that were so deeply rooted in my brain, causing me to have a real self-esteem problem. I was aware of everything that was happening in the room and of everything she was saying. After seven sessions, I was already feeling different. I succeeded in taking the final composure test and passed it.

But stress kept on coming back in my daily life, whether it was while facing an unexpected event or after having fought with someone I liked.

I am currently facing a situation where I must manage my stress and emotions, the latter of which are all over the place. I question myself, whether I will be able to succeed in doing so.

CHAPTER 2. SOME DREADFUL NEWS

24th of July 2018. A date that will stay engraved in my memory as the day that changed my life dramatically. It was the day the big fight started.

At 2.30 p.m., I hear my phone ring and a strange foreboding seizes me, as if I could sense what was going to happen next. I do not pick up the phone, I stand paralysed, feeling knots begin to twist in my stomach. I just stare at it while it continues to vibrate.

The strange feeling grows as I see the voicemail signal appear on my phone. When I eventually hear the voice of the gynaecologist, her tone and her words make me shiver:

"Good morning, I have just received the results of your biopsy, and unfortunately, they are not good. You will probably have to undergo surgery. I will check in with you when I come back. Everything is going to be alright. You can call your doctor. He has the results as well and will tell you more about them…"

She was actually closing her office to go on holidays when she called me. She would not have been able to reach out to me after, so she wanted to give me a proper follow-up before leaving. She wanted to give me the news herself. I found it really honourable. By now my body feels heavy, and I hear her words echoing in my head. I feel a weakness come over me.

My body starts shaking, and I begin crying uncontrollably. I try to pull myself together and decide to call the doctor. There must be a mistake. Time seems to be dragging. The phone rings and the secretary makes me wait for minutes that feel like hours…only for me to get knocked out a second time. The results are correct. We are talking about my breast, and about cancer. Crying and shaking, I sit down on the floor. My strength has left me, and I cannot hear anything anymore. It feels like I'm in a nightmare… it had neve even occurred to me that I might have to experience this feeling. I feel completely unprepared, caught by feelings I cannot really describe or put a finger on. The spectrum ranges from fear, anxiety, fright and doubt, to a lack of understanding and even anger.

My husband is asleep because he works night shifts. I cannot wait for him to wake up, it's too hard, I need to share this with him. I enter the room and sit down on the bed. He seems so still and calm, so far from imagining what is going on. I call his name gently. He wakes up startled and notices that I am crying.

"Hey, what's happening?" He asks.

"The gynaecologist has just called. She had my results and they were not good."

I would always remember the look he gave me, his sadness when he heard the news. He takes me in his arms immediately and we start crying together.

"I am scared…so scared", I say.

My teeth are chattering, my arms and legs are shaking. I cannot control my body. I am asking myself a thousand questions, but no answer comes to my mind.

"What did the gynaecologist tell you?"

"That it was not good and that I will have to undergo surgery. But then…is it cancer? Do you think that I have cancer? It is not possible… I'm having a bad dream."

"It's going to be alright. I love you honey," my husband replies.

My body is out of control. It belongs to someone else. I am shaking, I feel like vomiting. My stomach is in pain, I'm having an out-of-body experience, as if I were just watching the scene from afar. It is such a weird and terrifying feeling. I am bewildered and panic-stricken by the whole thing. The very same night, we have an appointment at the doctor. We have to find someone to look after the children because I don't want them to be aware of what's going on. I eventually decide to call my parents. I already know how much pain and fear I am going to cause them. It frightens me even more. My mum picks up the phone:

"Hi sweetie! How are you?"

"I'm fine. Well…actually, not really. Can you put the phone on speaker so that Dad can hear me please?"

A loud noise is banging in my head. I feel nauseous and have a lump in my throat.

"Okay, you're on speaker," my mother answers "what is wrong dear?"

I explain the situation to them while trying to remain calm. It is hard and I feel their pain over the phone. But they keep their composure and remain positive.

We do not know much for the moment, it will be clearer tonight. Waiting for the verdict, I try to keep my head cool. My eyes meet my husband's, who himself looks devastated.

CHAPTER 3. CONFIRMATION FROM THE DOCTOR

It really is a bomb that has just exploded at home, but we will have to remain calm as I don't want to worry the children.

It is 4.30 p.m., they are waking up and I do not want to stress them out. I wipe my tears and try to breathe calmly. I need to put on a mask, I can't show them how scared I'm feeling. Here we go. My husband is being very helpful. He too is worrying, but he is trying not to show anything either.

I give them a snack while trying to put on a calm and smiling face. I cannot wait to see the doctor and to have some answers. A lot of questions are flying through my head, and I still feel like I'm in a bad movie. This can't actually be happening, could it?

At 5.45 p.m., we arrive at my parents', who live ten minutes away from us. I take a deep breath before getting out of the car. I do not want to increase their sense of worry. I realise immediately that my parents are actually doing the same. Somehow that reassures me. Are we responding the right way though? I do not know.

Is it some kind of protection for us all? Probably.

It is 6 p.m. and we are entering the doctor's waiting room. I'm holding my husband's hand. I'm shaking again but I manage to control it a bit better this time. A man is sitting in front of us, another to our left. When our eyes meet, I have the feeling that they know why I am here, as if the word 'cancer' was engraved on my forehead. My phone rings, I pick up and hear the voice that had made me shiver earlier. My gynaecologist wants to talk to me before she leaves. She had taken my phone number to call me from the airport. She apologises for telling me what was happening so abruptly and explains to me that she did not want to go on holidays abroad for ten days without giving me the results. She thought that it would have been unprofessional. I thank her sincerely, because even though her message was a shock, her empathy and devotion to explain the results to me, moved me. I understand how she felt perfectly. She then tells me that I will probably have to undergo surgery but that all the steps will be carefully monitored. Everything was going to be alright.

I feel reassured even though the situation does not seem much clearer to me. I go back to the waiting room and tell everything about the conversation to my husband. The doctor comes into the room. My legs are heavy, I am hot. I feel really weak.
At last, I am going to have some answers. Which kind of surgery? When? Where? Am I going to need chemotherapy? Is it bad? Could I die?

She explains part of the situation to me. The same words always come back: cancer, tumour, specialist, surgery. She has already called the oncology centre that is situated one hour away from our house and I have an appointment next Monday, on the 29th of January. I will meet with the oncologist, the surgeon, and one of the social workers. Some additional medical exams might be needed so we will have to stay for the day. It's going to be a long journey. I have to be strong and courageous.

She puts me on sick leave, it's difficult for me to accept that. I do not feel sick, so to just stop working so suddenly for an unknown time period makes me incredibly sad. I will not have enough time to prepare myself psychologically to part with the children I am taking care of. It all seems sudden, difficult and abnormal. Not just for me but also for my own children who are so used to them, to being with them. The bond between us had grown strong quite quickly. Their parents are going to have to find another playschool assistant and quickly as well. The children will have to get used to new rules, to a new house. It will be difficult for them, and I feel responsible for it. The doctor states that I will have to stay on a sick leave for at least a year, which seems like such a long time.

I spend the weekend waiting with my doubts and questions, time seems to be dragging. However, I try to enjoy the present moment with my husband and my children. Time seems suspended in the air. It is a very strange sensation.

The night from Sunday to Monday seems short. I'm agitated and have many nightmares.

CHAPTER 4. THE ONCOLOGY CENTRE

By the time of the appointment, I'm actually feeling quite calm, my husband is by my side. We are eager to know more about what lies ahead.

A door opens and a man wearing white scrubs calls my name. What should I expect? Is it bad? Is it too late? So many questions start buzzing around in my head again.

We enter, I'm a bit more tensed now. We are introduced to an oncologist and a social worker. I can feel my stress level is increasing now. I feel like I'm in a bubble. People talk to me, but I cannot understand or even hear most of what I am told. The man who opened the door is the surgeon. He examines me by feeling my left breast. He can feel the two lumps very clearly. My other breast seems fine. Nothing under my armpits either. I put my clothes back on.

We then talk about my medical history, as well as about my family's. We also discuss my family life. My pregnancies. It's a long Q & A session.

He explains to me that I will have to undergo a mammography and that I'll see him again when the results come back. He will explain everything then.

The secretary escorts us all the way to the exam department and asks us to wait for a short while. It is the first time that I have to do a mammography. I know the theory but am still wondering what it is in practice and above all, what the result is going to be.

A woman comes towards me. I have to follow her and to undress myself to the waist. A bit confused, I walk towards the machine. The woman, probably in her thirties, is sweet and calm and puts me at ease immediately. The exam starts. The machine pushes against my breast. I feel oppressed but breathe calmly until the end. My breast, ribs and shoulders are hurting now. The machine comes closer to me, time now gets slower. Eventually it is over. The soothing voice of the young lady tells me to go back to the surgeon's waiting room.

The door is slightly open, the surgeon is already waiting for us. I hand him the documents I was given. He looks at them thoroughly, taking his time. I am trying to read his gaze. A sudden fear grabs me. After a few long minutes, he eventually says:

"Your breasts are too dense. There are some dark areas, but I cannot see properly," he goes on. "You will have to undergo an MRI scan before the surgery, for us not to miss anything."

I do not know what to answer. He continues:

"You are very young, we will hit this cancer hard. I will start with a surgery called a lumpectomy, to withdraw the two tumours. You'll be able to keep your breast."

At hearing the news, I smile spontaneously. He carries on:

"You will probably have to go through chemotherapy and radiotherapy; We'll know more about it after the surgery, as we'll take samples to analyse the tumours and adapt the treatment as much as possible. At the moment, you have what we call a Stage 2 Cancer."

Stages go from 0 to 5. I am relieved that my cancer is not at a higher stage, but cannot help thinking that a Stage 2 is already pretty bad.

"Alright," I answer still a bit voiceless.

"We are going to set a date for the surgery together. So…there is some availability on the 7th of February."

I feel my heart miss a beat. Laughing nervously I reply:

"The 7th of February? That early? But that's next week."

He smiles at me and confirms.

"It's a bit too early, I don't feel ready" I say still smiling nervously.

"I understand," he says. "What about the 20th then?"

"It works for me…"

The date is now set. It is stressful but at the same time, I cannot wait to get rid of these tumours and to start the fight.

We keep on talking. He gives us more explanations, we go through more Q&A sessions, and we set more medical appointments: mammary MRI, anaesthetist, heart scintigraphy, bone scintigraphy and other specialists.

He also asks me if we were planning on having a baby in the future. My eyes meet my husband's and we smile at each other. I answer:

"Yes, but not immediately."

He then explains that undergoing chemotherapy might make me sterile. He offers to carry out an egg preservation procedure, in order to freeze my eggs and save them for future use. We decide we are going to think about it. It is a whole new area to contemplate.

CHAPTER 5. A REVEALING EXAMINATION

The following days almost seem normal. I do not feel sick. Cancer is so insidious. It lies right in our core, but we are not aware of its presence, we cannot feel it. This disease is invisible. But in spite of everything, I succeed in staying positive.

Telling my family and friends that I am sick is very difficult. I do not really feel sorry for myself, but I am afraid to sadden other people. Usually, as soon as I tell people, I can sense a strong emotion in their eyes and in their voice.

On the 12th of February, I have to undergo the mammography. I am calm about it and do not ask myself any questions. It only is an additional clarification for the surgeon, so nothing to worry about.

The examination goes fine and at the end of it, I am asked to go to the waiting room, as a doctor wants to see me. It immediately arouses my curiosity, as in each room, there are posters informing patients that the results would be given at a later stage.

I wait for a while, I have to be patient which isn't something I'm particularly good at.

The doctor arrives and asks me to show her the precise location of the two lumps in my breast. I show her. She looks at them, touches them. I am starting to wonder what is going on. She explains:

"We can see a dark zone appears on the MRI, that's separate from the lumps we already know about. It could mean that there is a cancerous area in your lower breast that would change the type of operation you have to undergo."

I remain speechless. I was so calm and now I am starting to worry. I bite the bullet and answer:

"Might you have to remove the whole breast?"

"I cannot tell you right now, I will have to schedule an ultrasound scan. I see that you already have an appointment with the anaesthetist the day after tomorrow in the afternoon, so would you be available tomorrow morning?"

I cannot make up my mind. It is an hour away from home, I would have to stay there the whole day. However, I do not really have the choice and agree to make the appointment.

"Will I know more after the scan then?"

"You will," she says. "The scan will be more accurate, we will know exactly where the tumours are."

"You are stressing me out Doctor," I reply, laughing nervously.

She apologises, smiles and continues:

"Do not worry. For the moment, we cannot make any definitive statement."

After this appointment, I do not feel reassured at all. I meet again with the same taxi driver who drove me there. On the drive home we talk about my situation very openly and plainly. I actually found it very helpful.

I want to underline that I really enjoyed all the trips back and forth with the taxi drivers. They don't just drive us to our medical exams. The follow our entire journey, they know when to engage with us and when to remain silent. Empathy, respect, attentiveness, they have the interpersonal qualities that enhance our well-being.

It's the 14th of February at last, the day of the scan. I am nervous and one question sticks in my mind: 'Is it worse than expected?' I'm hoping to find out soon. A cheerful lady carries out the scan. She is looking at the screen while I am staring at her. She does not say a word, does not move a jot. I decide to look at the screen as well, but it does not help. Shadows and dark spots. Is it normal? I feel my heart quiver.
She doesn't say anything.
Eventually, she says:

"Sit down please, I will explain to you."
It makes me shudder and I can already feel tears in my eyes. I sit down and listen.

"The two first scans showed two lumps in the middle of your breast. The MRI, on the other hand, also showed a dark zone in the lower part of it, as does the scan you have just undergone. The surgeon will talk to you, but you probably will have to undergo a mastectomy."

I feel the tears rolling down my cheeks and answer:

"I understand. I will have to fight against this cancer. I had not imagined that, but it will be alright."

"It is better to withdraw the whole breast, to make sure that nothing bad remains. The surgeon will tell you everything. He will see you today, he has a slot available between two patients."

I dry my tears and take a deep breath.

While putting my clothes back on, I feel deeply shaken and deeply indifferent at the same time. Two contradictory emotions. The stress goes up and down in waves, as if my mind was processing the fact that it is the best solution.

From this day on, I keep on repeating to myself 'my breast for my life'. The motto reassures, strengthens me, and helps me face what is going to happen next.

CHAPTER 6. CHANGE OF PLAN

It is now lunch time. I sit down in the cafeteria and think back on everything that happened. Words echo in my head. The scenes go by. I need to build up my strength.

While eating, I tell my sister in arms, Sophie, about my appointment and how I feel about it. She is someone I love dearly. She understands me, as she went through the same disease. She is a real driving force for me.

We met on Facebook. We were part of the same playschool assistant group. When I had to stop working, I was a bit confused with all the paperwork to fill in and she helped me out, gave me many good pieces of advice. Then, she often checked in with me and we stayed in touch. She ended up becoming a friend. A real cornerstone of my new life. I will never thank her enough. She always knows what to say to push me forward, to make it easier to accept the situation. I know I can rely on her anytime.

It is time to call my parents and my brother to update them on the situation. I put myself back together until I feel serene, quite relaxed. I succeed in being in a good mood and even crack a joke.

I act the same towards my husband when he calls me, asking for some news. I feel good, in good hands.

Time goes by, I pass it anyway I can. At last it is time. The surgeon welcomes me in his office, reads the scan report and examines me again.

"There are two solutions," he starts. "Either we proceed to a mastectomy, that is to say that we will remove the breast. It will be possible to consider a reconstruction later. Or we can keep a small part of the breast, the upper part. Given the state of the tissues, we would need to have a healthy leeway, otherwise you might have to undergo surgery twice. It would not be very aesthetic, but it is yours to think about it and to decide."

I answer immediately:

"The complete removal. I prefer to do it in one go, instead of taking the risk of going through a second surgery. Besides, it seems more aesthetic anyway."

He smiles at me with compassion, puts his hand on my shoulder and tells me:

"You are very courageous and you are making the right decision. It is not mine to decide but I think that it is the safest choice."

I smile back at him and feel that my cheeks are wet.

"Thank you, I keep on telling myself that it is 'my breast for my life."

"And you are right..."

The surgery is still set for the 20th of February. I have one week to get ready for a change of physical appearance. The taxi driver comes and picks me up. I do not talk much, I am lost in my thoughts.

When I arrive at home, I immediately gaze at my husband. He is sitting on the couch. He looks sad and disconnected. I come closer to him, take him in my arms and whisper that everything is going to be alright.

"I am afraid to lose you," he confesses.

"Do not think about it. I will not die, I am pretty confident about it."

He answers with glistening eyes:

"I know, but anything could happen."

We hold each other tenderly, whispering sweet words, trying to make the other feel better.

My husband is scared to lose me. Even if I understand why, I do not share his negative thoughts. I cannot afford to think this way. We have to be strong, positive and confident. And actually, it is just how I feel.

At night-time, my body becomes unmanageable: tremors, stomach aches, nauseas, as if I was going through the whole acceptation process again. My head fills up with questions. Will my relationship be strong enough to go through this? How can I look at myself and accept my body with only one breast?

I go to bed early in order to forget about everything.

Little by little, I come to terms with the situation. I look at pictures as often as possible not to be shocked when I will wake up on the day of the surgery.

In the meantime, I enjoy my family life. I live and behave as usual. With my husband, we agree to explain everything to the children. However, sometimes, words do not come easily. We are afraid to scare them. Days go by and we procrastinate. The day of the surgery is approaching quickly, we will tell them after. They already know that I am undergoing surgery, that I am very sick and that the doctors will do everything in their power to cure me. We can tell them about the rest later.

CHAPTER 7. 'MY BREAST FOR MY LIFE'

The first round is about to start. I put my gloves and my helmet on, getting ready for the fight. My husband comes with me. They get us set up in a prep room, we will have to wait a bit.

A nurse comes and takes my vitals, blood-pressure, temperature and so on. She also checks my personal information. She asks me to put on a pair of scrubs and slippers.

I joke around with my husband, and he takes a picture of me in my very sexy outfit. I do not think too much about what is going to happen. I feel ready and relaxed.

A member of the staff comes in, it's time to identify the sentry ganglion. I get injected with a radioactive product that is supposed to tint the ganglion blue. It will allow the surgeon to proceed to a ganglionic D and C during the surgery if needed.

The product is directly injected into my breast. It stings, I can feel it spreading, the nurse massages me to soothe the effect.

I go back to my room and wait until it's time for the surgery. When the porter arrives, I feel overcome suddenly with emotion. I kiss my husband and follow the porter with a knot in my stomach.

I end up in a small waiting room and a nurse comes to me. She explains to me how the surgery will unfold and sets me up on a small bed. Several nurses are now moving around me.

They measure my blood-pressure and connect me to a catheter. A real scrubs parade is taking place in the room.

It is too much pressure for me, and I start crying uncontrollably. I panic, my body starts shaking, my nerves are breaking down.

The nurses do everything they can to take my mind off the whole thing, but it is difficult. Even if they are taking extra-care of me, I am focused on the upcoming surgery.

Is it going to be alright? How am I going to react when I will see myself with only one breast? Is it going to hurt? Am I going to wake up?

The surgeon comes closer to me and, noticing my behaviour, puts his hand on my arm gently and tries to reassure me.

I am guided to the operating room. I already feel better and my smile comes back, as well as my good mood. I even joke around with the nurses.

They put a mask on my face. I have to count until ten. 1, 2, 3, 4… I fall asleep and the surgery can start.

A few hours later, I come to and discover that I am in the recovery room. Everything is blurry, I can hear voices but cannot understand what they are talking about. I try to move but fall back asleep. It happens several times in a row before I eventually wake up from my deep sleep.

A nurse comes to me:

"The surgery went well, and you are in the recovery room. How do you feel?"

"I feel alright but my left arm hurts," I answer with a weak voice.

"It is normal. The sentry ganglion was reached, and the surgeon had to proceed to a ganglionic D and C. We gave you pain killers, the pain should be numbed soon."

"Thank you."

As soon as she leaves, I put my hand on my breast. It is flat. I raise my head slightly and have a look. I am wearing a scrub so I cannot see anything. But I still can see that a part of me is missing. No reaction, no tears. I accept the situation. Even better: I feel relieved to have uprooted this cancer.

I am delighted to find my husband waiting for me in my room. He seems well, stirred with emotion, but well. I spend a lot of time sleeping, the surgery tired me. The rest of the day, as well as the night, go by normally.

The next morning, a nurse comes to withdraw my drip. It is a relief, as it is painful and impairing my movement.

I have to go take a shower but my whole body hurts now. I am so stiff. I slowly reach the bathroom.

I undress myself, and spontaneously look at my reflection in the large mirror that has been calling me. I take a deep breath and raise my head.

A strange feeling grasps me. A strong emotion threatens to overwhelm me, but I control it. A huge plaster hides the scar on my breast. And another one goes is located under my armpit.

It is so flat. Half of my body looks like a man's body. I keep on repeating to myself: 'my breast for my life'.

Then it is time to go back home. I get ready. Two ambulance drivers take me to my house.

I am delighted to go back to my family. Besides, I can handle the pain thanks to the medication.

The next day, I am supposed to bring my daughter to school. I need to do it, I want to face the reaction of other people right now, as I don't know whether I will have the courage to do so if I wait for too long. When you fall from a horse, you have to go back on it immediately. I was doing the same. Looking back on it, it was a bit reckless. I needed to sleep above anything else.

I had asked my mum to come with me because I was fairly weak.

A nurse regularly comes home to change my plasters. My bruises are huge and very sensitive. But I'm in a good mood and intend on staying as such!

CHAPTER 8. ANATOMOPATHOLOGY

Three weeks later, on the 7th of March, I have an appointment scheduled with the surgeon. I couldn't wait to know more about my tumours, be careful what you wish for.

My husband was able to take some time off work to come with me. I'm confident. The surgeon looks at my scar. It looks healthy and clean. I will soon start the physiotherapy sessions to make it more flexible and to be able to move my arm again. The ganglionic D and C triggered much pain and stiffness. The physiotherapy will help me ease the pain.

We get down to business, the results of the analyses are ready. The surgeon starts:
"We had spotted two tumours and a cancerous zone in the lower part of your breast. Thanks to the analyses, we discovered that there were actually nine tumours spread throughout your breast. They measured between one and fifteen millimetres, while the cancerous zone was as big as eight centimetres."

"Gosh…" I reply, bewildered. "If I had not had that gynaecological appointment, I would have missed the whole thing."

"Yes, and it would have been much worse. The first ganglion had metastases and two others had micro-metastases. I hence withdrew seventeen ganglions, which means that your cancer is a Stage 3 Cancer now."

I am shocked. It was more than time to find out about this cancer, and to start fighting it.

He keeps on going:

"You made the right choice in choosing the mastectomy because what would have been left of your breast would not have been healthy."

I am relieved and ask:

"I will have to go through chemotherapy, won't I?"

"Indeed. You will undergo chemo and radiotherapy. Your tumours reacted to hormones, so you will also go through hormone therapy to avoid a relapse. It is a pill that you will have to take once a day. If your body adapts to it well, you will take it for the next ten years. Once every three weeks during an eighteen-month-period, you will go through Herceptin injections as well. It is a targeted therapy aimed at avoiding the proliferation of cancerous cells. Your heart will also be monitored regularly."

"It is a long treatment."

"Yes, but it is needed. You should tell yourself that the year to come will be a year off."

He is right. What lies ahead is a real obstacle course. One obstacle after the other, I will succeed though.

The following days, I had to go through a pelvic abdominothoracic scan and a bone scintigraphy. It was tough, part of the machine came as close to my face as possible. I had a feeling that it was going to crush me. I tried to remain calm, closed my eyes and took a deep breath. It was such a relief when I was told that there was no metastasis left.

On March the 26th, I meet with the oncologist. She explains to me what the chemotherapy is going to consist of three cycles of FEC 100, one every three weeks. Then, one treatment of Taxol every week for twelve weeks. The Herceptin injections will start at the same time as the Taxol.

On the 3rd of April, I take a DNA test to know if I carry a gene that would favour the development of cancer. I give a sample of my saliva and take a blood test. The results will be ready in a year. I will need to be patient.

I also met with a gynaecologist specialised in the conservation of oocytes (my eggs). I had to take daily injections of a product that stimulates ovulation. Then, I needed to do some more blood tests and ultrasound scans every two or three days to monitor the growth of the oocytes. It was a very stressful and painful process. The exams, were supposed to take eleven days, ended up taking around two weeks, the time it took for my oocytes to be ready to be sampled. I confess that at a point, I was on the brink of giving up. I was tired of medical appointments, fed up with injections. I was already thinking about the upcoming chemotherapy.

But I psyched myself up, it was important for both my husband and myself. We had to look towards the future.

The intervention went as planned. I was operated under local anaesthesia and had to take sedatives. They were able to freeze eleven of my oocytes. It gives us a good chance if we ever need it. Another thing done!

The day after, on the 6th of April, I had to undergo surgery…again. They had to install a PAC under my skin, a small case linked to a catheter, thin pipe slipped into a vein. I was again under local anaesthesia, and it was quick and painless.

However, it remained sensitive for several days after. I had the feeling I had a rubber-band in my neck. However, I am now used to living with this unknown object that is going to be part of me for a while.

I used to struggle to deal with the unknown, I now do not have the choice. Every single examination is different. Thanks to all of this, I am learning to manage my stress. Staying calm under any circumstance is delightful. A strong fate in myself and in the future gives me wings. I have everything I need to overcome all the obstacles in my way.

My relatives are surprised because they did not expect me to react this way. I understand, as I didn't either.

CHAPTER 9. SECOND ROUND

I knew from the beginning that I was going to lose my hair because of chemotherapy. I am getting psychologically ready. As a woman, it is unthinkable to imagine oneself bald. I have always had long hair. That is why I decide to go to the hairdresser to cut my hair short before it falls.

I choose a haircut with one side longer than the other, so that my relatives can get used step by step to the upcoming change.

Since I have learnt that I am sick, I have not been hiding anything from my children. They are aware of each step. When we talk about my upcoming hair loss, they laugh about it because they do not realise what it means. One night, I decide to show them a picture of a woman going through the same treatment as me.
I call them:

"My darlings, come here! I have to show you something…"
They rush towards me. I tell them:

"You know, I am going to lose my hair soon. I will wear scarves and beanies instead. I will show you a picture so that you can see."

They look at each other and laugh together. I show them:

"See, this woman lost all her hair, and soon I will as well."

My daughter states immediately:

"Oh! This is what 'not having hair' looks like. It is ugly."

Her smile had turned into surprise. As for my son, he does not say a word.

Of course, it hurts to hear my daughter's words, but I understand why she said so. The way they both pictured a bald person was flawed.

I continue with a smile:

"I will, of course, look different. But you know, it is not the disease that is going to make me lose my hair, but the cure. And it is very important that I take the medicine properly in order to heal completely. Besides, my hair will grow back quickly, you will see."

They nod, smiling, and go back to their games.

I am relieved to have shown them, to have prepared them for what was to come.

A few days later, to prepare them even more to see me with a scarf on my head, I start a fun activity. Each one of us has to take a scarf and tie it on the top of his or her head. To them, we look like Aladdin. We have a lot of fun taking pictures of each other and parading through the whole house. It would create great memories when everything would be over, and we would all laugh about it. It also makes the situation lighter, so I am definitely enjoying it.

It's the 9th of April and it is my first session of chemotherapy. The second round is about to start. Surprisingly enough, I am not worried. On the contrary, I am quite serene. It is not like me, but I embrace the zen like attitude with pleasure.

My mother is with me. I am in a single room for now. The nurse tells me that there are rooms shared by two or three people. I like the idea of being together and being able to share our story.

She is really nice and sweet and explains everything to me. I trust her.

She puts the perfusion in my PAC. The patch supposed to kill the pain that was installed an hour before is effective, I do not feel anything.

She also gives me products that kill the pain brought about by chemotherapy. I take an anti-vomiting tablet as well, will have to take it again over the next two days.

Then comes the chemotherapy itself. Two long syringes of a bright red liquid. This poison flows into my body, but without it, I cannot heal. That is why I take it, accept it.

The nurse explains to me which kind of side effects I could have during the following hours, or even days. She repeats the endless list I was already given some days ago. Nausea, vomiting, tiredness, hair loss… I could go on.

I listen to her very carefully, but I do not want to overthink what is to come either, so I tell myself that I might not have any symptom at all. We will see.

The first treatment goes as planned. I feel good. A few hours later, the nurse unplugs me and wishes me luck.

The very moment I get up from the bed, I realise how weak and nauseous I am. My skin is pale. I reassure my mother who is worried about me and we go back home.

Tiredness seizes my body and mind for four days. I really have to motivate myself to bring my daughter to school every day and to take care of my son during the day. Their presence lifts me up though.

I also take advantage of the fact that my son takes daily naps and I do the same.

Each time I wake up, my furred mouth ruins my appetite. But I don't feel nauseous. It is a small victory. I am relieved to be able to handle the treatment this well.

Fifteen days later, I will be disillusioned.

CHAPTER 10. BALD

This morning, when I put my fingers in my hair, a handful stays in my hands. How awful. It does not matter how much I have been preparing for it, the image is still terrible. One more time, I put my fingers in my hair to make sure it is real. To my utter disappointment, more hair comes out. I'm already imagining shaving my head.

I watch pictures and videos on the internet to find ideas and pieces of advice.

We are currently moving into a new house, so I am mentally and physically tired. It is not the right time. I am overwhelmed by my emotions and cannot stop crying when I'm annoyed at something.

I call to make an appointment with the hairdresser. She could see me in thirty minutes. I am simultaneously sure of my decision and terrified about it.

I arrive in the salon and sit down in an armchair while waiting for her to be done with one of her customers.

While I am watching her, I feel a knot forming in my stomach. My heart beats faster and faster, I am completely lost in my thoughts.

I jump off my chair and tell her:

"I'm not ready. I cannot shave my head today. It is not an easy situation, I'm sorry."

I start shedding a tear.

"I completely understand. I can offer you a very short haircut instead if you would like. It would be less of a shock and you would have more time to get ready."

Let's do this, it seems like a good compromise. I leave the salon with a smile on my face and five centimetres of hair on my head. I look like a boy but at least, I still have my hair.

Unfortunately, three days later, some holes start forming in my hair. I cannot postpone it this time and will have to shave my head.

This step is very difficult. I reluctantly make the appointment. But when the hairdresser eventually shaves my head, I feel relieved. I did it! I am kind of proud of myself. I feel strong and victorious.

When I come back home with a beanie on my head, I am afraid about what my husband is going to think. I put myself in his shoes, or at least I try to do so. Seeing his wife without hair must be quite shocking and disturbing.

I come back home, my husband gives me an uneasy smile and his eyes become wet when I remove the beanie. I hold him in my arms immediately. It is a huge step for the two of us, but our love will come out stronger. I am positive about it. I trust our relationship.

The following days, I get used to my new appearance and so does my family. I wear beanies, coloured scarves, large earrings and some make-up. I kind of like my new look and accept myself as I am.

My husband does not change his attitude either and still desires me. I am his wife, and nothing is going to change this. His love lifts me up and gives me the strength to handle the situation.

How lucky I am to have him by my side!

It is already time for the second course of chemotherapy. I am fully motivated and ready to face it.

Everything goes as planned. The nurses are very kind, and so are my roommates. The side effects are a bit harder to deal with but are still bearable. A sore appears on my gum. It's a nagging pain and eating becomes difficult, so I try out everything that could soothe my pain: gel, homeopathy tablets... It will take time, but it will pass.

During the third round, I start feeling nauseous. Since I've learnt that I had cancer, I have lost five kilos and am getting increasingly tired. I have to take naps more regularly. New mouth sores come out before I can even get rid of the others.

I start losing both my common sense and my memory, simple things become difficult, and some daily gestures are not as spontaneous as they used to be. I have to focus not to make mistakes. It is very disturbing, and I feel kind of lost at times.

But it is such a relief to be done with these three rounds of chemo. Another step is over, and I am proud of myself.

I will now be able to start the other treatments, once a week. It is going to be a new rhythm, with new symptoms, but step by step I am getting closer to being cured.

CHAPTER 11. MY CHILDREN

My six-year-old daughter has been nervous for a few days now. I cannot tell her anything without making her shout or cry. Whether at school or at home, it is starting to become complicated. I decide to get in touch with a community service which works remotely with the Breast Cancer Treatment Organisation. I learned that I could benefit from psychological assistance and so could my children.
I make an appointment for my daughter some days later.

At lunch time, while eating, I explain to her:
"We are going to go see a woman together and talk to her."
"To talk about your disease?" She answers curtly.
"Exactly, but to talk about you as well because you seem to be going through a rough time."
Knocking her fist on the table and giving me a dirty look, she screams:
"I knew it. You are not telling me everything!"
I feel disconcerted, but I keep it to myself and answer quickly:

"Of course we are darling, why would you say such a thing? I have explained everything to you, but this woman can help you accept the situation and better understand it. Do you have any other questions?"

"No. I understood everything."

"Are you sure? Because you can ask me anything…"

"I know."

"You know that my hair is going to grow back?"

"Yes, you told me."

"And you also know that the doctors are doing the best they can to help me."

"I know."

"Do you want to know anything else? Feel free to ask me any question."

"Where did they put your sick breast?"

Well, I was not expecting this type of question. I ask back:

"What do you think? Where did they put it?"

"In the bin of the hospital?" She asks.

"Exactly, in the bin. It was very sick."

With a big smile on her face, she keeps on chatting while finishing her meal, her sweet voice sounding joyful again.

From then on, my little girl was back. I do not know what she had imagined, but it was definitely time to talk about the situation again. From the beginning, I had been telling them everything, but she still believed the contrary.

She spoke calmly with the psychologist who concluded that everything was back to normal, thanks to the verbalisation of the problem. And indeed, at home, everything is back to normal.

My son is probably too young to understand everything going on. However, he always needs to know where I go, why, and above all, if I will come back. I do my best to reassure my children, in order for them to be at ease, and so that the situation is not too much of a burden for them.

Today, we have to go to the phone shop. Once there, we talk to the woman in charge about the various options we could choose from to be able to enjoy the internet in our new home.
My son, who is sitting next to me, takes advantage of a break in the conversation to throw spontaneously:

"You are missing a breast!"
Quite embarrassed, I try to ignore him but the inevitable happens:

"Mummy! You only have one breast!"
I look at him and tell him:

"Shush! Listen to the lady please!"
Obviously, my answer does not satisfy him, but it's not the right time to discuss it.
While leaving the shop, I tell him:

"You know, people do not need to be aware that mummy is sick, and that one of my breasts is missing. It will be our secret."

Children are spontaneous and natural, so he will probably do it again. I cannot resent him, even if it is very embarrassing.

CHAPTER 12. CHEMOTHERAPY: PART II

After having gone through my first three rounds of heavy chemotherapies, I will now have to go through twelve more. It is going to be a different product though, Taxol, which is likely to bring about different side effects as well.

After the first injection, I will have to stay a few hours under surveillance, to make sure that I am not intolerant to the product.

The good news is that the product is not supposed to trigger nausea. Nevertheless, it can trigger pins and needles in your hands and feet, a fact that I would figure out soon enough.

As for the Herceptin, the targeted therapy, it will start at the same time. My heart will be monitored very carefully during the entire treatment period, with ultrasound scans every three months. Then, the scans will take place every six months for twenty-four months following the treatment, and every year for five years afterwards.

I handle the two new products quite well, and discover little by little that I can be very dynamic. Unfortunately, things become a bit more complicated half-way through the cure.

The side effects start lasting three to four days after each injection. Shivers, headaches, body stiffness…

I get pins and needles as well as a burning feeling in my hands and also in my feet. The pain is unbearable, whether I am walking or just sitting down.

After the ninth round, they decide to decrease the dose of chemotherapy so that the treatment would be more comfortable for me.

However, I am still motivated and eager to be done with it.

Before every session, I have to see a doctor, and he or she has to approve the treatment. Then I go to a room and get started.

On the 21st of August, my tenth round is cancelled because of the strong neuropathic pain I am undergoing, even if the dose itself is not as high as it should be. The week before the decision to cancel, I had lost both my strength and sensitivity. I had started to drop objects without even realising it. It felt strange.

The doctor had then got in touch with the oncologist and asked for a second opinion and, unfortunately, they both agreed on cancelling the tenth round, as they did not want to take any risks.

It is a hard blow for me. They try to reassure me by saying that a week break could help the symptoms to improve, and hence allow me to take the two last injections.

I go to the room where I will get the injection of Herceptin, that has been given the green light. My roommate is very friendly. We talk about our lives, about the treatments, and of course about cancer. It is really enjoyable to feel understood. She finishes my sentences and vice-versa. We have the same mindset and the same strategy to fight against this disease that touches so many people. I almost forget about the earlier disappointment.

It is not always like this. I have also met people who did not want to talk about it, and of course, it is theirs to decide and I have to accept it. Once, I met a woman who was about to undergo her first chemotherapy. She was very nervous, so we talked a lot and she eventually felt better.

Towards the end of my treatment, I came across a seventy-five-year-old woman coming for her first round as well. She was very upset by what was happening to her and burst into tears each time a nurse was approaching her. It was more difficult. Even though I was going through the same thing, I did not really know what to say.

Actually, what would be 'the right thing' to say? We are all different and so are our reactions.

The eleventh round goes very smoothly. I'm glad to be able to get back in the ring. Even if the dosage of product is still diminished, I am moving forward and am starting to see the light at the end of the tunnel.

CHAPTER 13. AN UNFORESEEN EVENT

Today is my mother's birthday. I feel weak and very tired. I keep it to myself and get ready because my parents invited us to come to their place to celebrate.

As soon as we arrive, the colour of my face makes them worry about me.

I reassure them:

"I just feel a bit tired, it will not last."

However, I do not have any appetite. I cannot even finish my meal and have to skip dessert because of a nagging stomach-ache. I am getting increasingly tired, increasingly weak.

I really try not to show it too much, as it is not the moment to be sick. But my parents have already started to worry anyway, so we decide to measure my blood-pressure. My mother has a blood-pressure monitor at home to check on her hypertension.

My blood pressure seems fine, 11/5, but my heart rate reaches up to 98 BPM while at rest. It is probably due to my levels of stress and tiredness. Hours go by and I feel worse and worse, to a point where I even get nausea and diarrhoea.

My heart rate now reaches 115 BPM. My family and I agree to call the emergency services, thinking that they are going to reassure me.

The doctor tells me that I will have to go to the emergency room. They will have to carry out an ECG to understand my condition. The fact that they tell me to come immediately also increases my stress level. It is 5 p.m. and tomorrow morning, it is my children's first day in their new school. Another reason to be anxious, as I am still hoping to be back home tonight.

The journey seems endless, and I now have the feeling that a knife is stabbing my chest. When we arrive, we are surprised to see so many people there. There are patients on stretchers everywhere, as well as people waiting to be taken care of. Someone takes care of me immediately, I need to lie down. They take my blood-pressure, my heart rate and my temperature and I am then told that the wait could be as long as four hours. My constants are normal, except for my heart rate. A nurse asks me:

"Do you feel any pain in your chest?"

"A bit from time to time," I answer spontaneously.

"Alright. You will have to wait for a doctor to be available in order to carry out an ECG."

Half an hour later, nothing has improved. I am still tired and weak. I feel an acute pain in my chest. I tell the nurse so that he can warn a doctor. Two nurses ask my husband to go out and make me undress myself to the waist. They look young and I am afraid to shock them with my half-man, half-woman chest. While undressing myself, I warn them that I underwent a mastectomy and it makes me feel better. To my great satisfaction, the ECG seems normal. I now have to wait to carry out other examinations.

At 7.30 p.m., it is time to get organised as far as the children are concerned, but there is almost no phone service at the hospital. My husband goes back home to get their clothes ready so that they can sleep at my parents'. A few minutes after he left, I am redirected to another section. A nurse takes a sample of my blood and I also have to do a urine test. Then, I have to wait again.

Around 9.30 p.m., the doctor comes to me and tells me that all the results are normal. My heart rate went back to normal as well and I am allowed to go back home. I will just have to call them if anything happens during the night.

I am so relieved. He explains to me that it might be due to the treatment and to the accumulation of tiredness.

I will be able to accompany my children to school tomorrow in the end. I'm not only relieved, but also delighted.

I sleep well and the next day, I feel great, as if nothing had happened.

A few days later, it is time for the twelfth & final round. I was already imagining myself being overjoyed, full of energy, and going around to thank people for their care.

I come down to Earth with a bang when the doctor tells me that I am not going to do it. I am still having symptoms. I am still dropping objects and I cannot open bottles anymore. On top of this, my heart condition reinforces his idea that he should cancel the last injection. I am disappointed, I did not go through the entire treatment.

My feelings are intermingled, half-way between disappointment and pride. Everything is muddled in my head.

I am delighted to be done with the chemo, bewildered to have missed the last one, and sad to say goodbye to the medical staff. They are part of our daily lives as patients, and we often develop kind of a relationship with them.

After the Herceptin cure, I give the nurses a box of chocolate to thank them.

They do an amazing job. They look after us, reassure us, give us the complementary information we need and listen to us.

From now on, I will have intramuscular injections of Herceptin at my house. Every three weeks. I'm over the moon.

CHAPTER 14. SHARING IS CARING

We are now in August, and I think about everything that has happened to me, everything I have had to go through. I think about the fight that I have been waging for the past six months. I think about all the women who are doing just the same, as there are so many of us, and about all the people suffering from any other type of cancer.

I was lucky to discover mine soon enough, but if I had known even sooner, the treatments would not have been as heavy. That is why I wanted to raise awareness among women, a wish that gave me the incentive to share my own experience on Facebook.

"To all the ladies,

It is important for me to share my struggle against the disease I am suffering from, because we all tend to think that it could never happen to us. But you never see it coming…

It is a routine gynaecological appointment that saved my life. An appointment that I almost cancelled.

My name is Mélanie, I am thirty-two, I am married and a mother of two. I was living a fulfilling life, that this gynaecological check-up turned upside-down when the doctor discovered two nodules in my breast. I was speechless. No one had ever had cancer in my family.

After several examinations, biopsies and a mastectomy, it turned out that I was suffering from a Stage 3 Cancer.

I could never thank my gynaecologist enough for having detected it and ensuring that I be taken care of as early as possible.

I am currently going through chemotherapy and will spare you the details. I will then have to undergo radiotherapy and hormone therapy.

When you learn about the disease, it is a shock, a nightmare.

You have to make appointments with one specialist after the other, and it goes so fast that the obstacle course starts quickly. The treatment procedure is triggered, and you have to follow it.

You go through the process day after day with strength and courage. But you sometimes do feel lonely, misunderstood by others.

No one can imagine what you are going through. Your fears, your doubts, your tiredness, your pain. Only people who have lived through it can understand.

Some friends grow apart, some acquaintances grow closer.

SO DON'T HESITATE:
- Go and see your gynaecologist regularly
- Check your breasts regularly

It does not take long and can save your life. When we are healthy, we tend to postpone such initiatives. On the internet, there is a lot of information about them.

***In order to convey the message to as many women as possible, thank you for sharing this publication!'

The publication was passed on one thousand four hundred times on Facebook and commented four hundred and eighty-four times. I am moved by the solidarity of the community. I really wanted to share, and I am delighted to have dared to do so.

After that, I had the honour to be contacted by 'We are patients' to talk about my experience. It is a French-speaking media that gives a voice to patients and patients' relatives who are committed to fight the disease.

Here is an excerpt from my testimony:

"What did the disease change in your life?"

"I used to be a 'worrier'. I was under so much pressure. Now I just go with the flow. I understood that the future could not be planned in detail and that we should enjoy the small daily pleasures."

"Did the disease strengthen your relationships with your loved ones?"

"It allowed me to realise who really cared about me: people I thought were real friends were not there for me as much as I was expecting them to be, whereas some acquaintances, work colleagues for example, were incredible.

I have also met a former 'fighter' online, a real warrior who gave me the weapons to fight against this cancer. She became very important for me, even if we only chat online, as we are living far away from each other.

I think that there are people who do not know how to react. And there are others who are in their bubble and do not even notice what we are going through. Thankfully, there are also the people who will always be there."

"How do you feel now?"

"I have always tried to keep a positive mindset and it has really helped me through. My family has been there for me the whole time as well. I have tried to do as many activities as I used to with my children, so that the situation would not be too much of a burden for them."

"Which piece of advice would you give to a patient?"

"If I could say something to the people going through the same hardship, and I know that there are still too many of us, it would be the following: 'Stay positive, hopeful, and combative. It will really help you to go through many things."

My testimony was shared two thousand one hundred and seventy-three times.

CHAPTER 15. RADIOTHERAPY

I am barely done with chemotherapy that I now have to start radiotherapy.

But little by little, I see the end of this obstacle race.

Before being able to start the radiotherapy sessions, an appointment is made in order to carry out a check-up. I am lying on my back, my arms raised above my head, and my head itself turned to the right. The table is hard and cold. It is uncomfortable, but it is a necessary evil.

The area that needs to be cured is scanned, and five points about the size of a needle are tattooed on my body. I have always wanted a tattoo! (Laughs)

The radiotherapist tells me that twenty-five sessions would be scheduled, at a pace of five a week, from Monday to Friday.

He also explains to me that I will always have to stay in the same position, and that I will stay in the room about fifteen minutes per session. The radiation time itself is only a few minutes long.

I will keep on seeing him once a week, to make sure that everything is going as planned.

I had agreed with the specialists that the radiotherapy be carried out in the hospital that is closest to my house, thirty kilometres away from it. Regarding the surgery and the chemotherapy, the doctor had given me no choice but to undergo them at a centre specialised in fighting cancer that was located an hour away from my place. As commuting was tiring, I now prefer being closer to my place to undergo the upcoming daily sessions.

Sessions go by very quickly and I have few side effects. No burning sensation and no red patches either. However, towards the end of the therapy, I feel my chest and my throat starting to tingle. It feels the same as a sore throat.

I am getting increasingly tired, the daily commutes and the lack of naps being partly responsible.

Today, on the 4th of October, I am getting ready for my first injection of Herceptin at home. I am delighted, I do not need to organize a babysitter for my children anymore and it is a real pleasure both for them, and for me.

When the nurse leaves, I feel extremely tired, depressed, and in a daze. I need to take a nap, I'm sure I will feel better afterwards. A few hours later, tremor, nausea and paleness appear. Is it normal? Maybe it's a once off, we'll see what happens next time I do it.

Unfortunately, the following sessions go down the same way, with a drop in my blood-pressure and heart rate. I know I still have a long way to go, and I feel that it is going to be difficult.

On the 9th of November, it is my last radiotherapy session and I am over the moon. I feel free and not compelled to commute to the hospital anymore. On the other hand, I feel left on my own and now quite passive in my fight against the disease.

I now can start taking the hormone therapy tablets, the treatment I will have to take daily for the next ten years to come. I hope that my body will cope well with it.

On the 20th of December, I meet with the oncologist again to do a recap. I thought that I had put on a bit of weight, but I did not know how right I was. When I climb onto the scale, what a surprise! I have put on six kilos in three months. The hormone therapy opened my appetite, and I have often been snacking in between meals lately. That will have to come to an end.

She asks me:

"How are the injections of Herceptin going?"

"Fine, but it is hard to get over them. It usually takes me a few days to do so. I cannot wait for it to be over."

"A few days? What are your symptoms?" She asks with surprise.

"My blood-pressure falls, so does my heart rate, and I feel particularly weak. The more I do it, the longer it takes to get over it. At the moment, it takes me about four days to feel better."

"I do not like that too much. I think that you will have to do it at the hospital again. It is possible that your body copes with the injections through the PAC better than it does with the ones through the muscles. Besides, at the hospital, we would be able to monitor your reactions."

"It is not that convenient for me though, I would have to reorganise everything as far as my children are concerned."

"I understand, but it is better. I do not want to take any risk as you don't seem to be tolerating it well. We usually inject it in thirty minutes, we will start by doing it in an hour and a half and see how it goes."

"Alright."

I am disappointed to probably have to go back to the centre every three weeks. It means that I would have to commute again, that I would waist precious time, and that I would have to get organised differently as far as school is concerned...nothing to look forward to.

But to be honest, I really don't feel good after the injections and it is then hard to cope with my children. The nurse measures my blood-pressure and my heart rate before each injection and comes back an hour after only to notice that they have decreased. It is not reasonable to keep on going like this. I really hope that I will tolerate the product better by going back to the hospital to carry on with the injections.

CHAPTER 16. RECONSTRUCTIVE SURGERY

I have already overcome a fair number of steps: the surgery, the chemotherapy and the radiotherapy. And six months from now, the Herceptin treatment will be over. Then a new obstacle race will start.

This January, I have another appointment with the surgeon, in order to talk about the different options I have regarding reconstructive surgery. I will not be able to start such a process before the end of the year though, as it is compulsory to wait for at least a year after the end of the radiotherapy.
The specialist gives me several options:

"We could put an expander in, it's a prothesis made of a deflated silicon envelope, that would be surgically installed. It would then be progressively filled up with physiological serum during consultations that would happen once or twice a week, until it reaches the right size. It would be replaced by a definitive prothesis three to four months later."

"Isn't it possible to install the prothesis directly and to skip the expander step?"

"No, because your skin would not be elastic enough. We can place the prothesis directly only when the reconstructive surgery is immediate, which is not your case because you underwent radiotherapy. The expander is used to elasticise the skin gradually."

"How long would the definitive prothesis last?"

"Between ten and fifteen years. You could also choose the biomodelling technique, for which we sample some fat from a chosen part of your body, and then use it to reconstruct your breast. It is carried out under general anaesthesia and you would have to do it in three or four stages. Then, another surgery would be needed to add the tattoo and the nipple. It would hence take around seven surgical interventions total if you were to choose this option."

"I wouldn't have thought it would be that long. So how long would it then take for the reconstruction to be completed ?"

"Let's say between a year and a year and a half according to the technique."

"Alright, I will have to think about it."

"Of course. We will see each other again in June. It will give you some time to think about it."

He hands a leaflet to me, in which there are plenty of details and pictures related to reconstructive surgery, and then continues:

"You did a DNA test for which we should have the results in a few months. We talked about it before, but if you carry a certain kind of gene, it is strongly advised, however not mandatory, to remove the other breast. The decision is yours."

"I remember, and my decision is already made, I do not want to take any risk. So if I carry a problematic gene, I prefer to have the other breast removed as well. My husband agrees with me."

"Perfect. You seem to be sure of your decision and you still think the same as the last time we saw each other. However, if we had to take such a measure, we would not be able to use the biomodelling technique. Given your build, I could only reconstruct one breast out of the two. You would have to use the expander."

He gives me an appointment for the month of May so that I can meet with a surgery nurse in order to talk some more about it, as well as another appointment to see him again in June.

I leave with a smile on my face, realising that I will have a woman's body again, my former body actually, the one I had missed so much. I would not have to think twice about what to wear anymore. Indeed, dressing up has been quite tough lately. If the cut is too low, it is obvious that a part of my body is missing, if it is too loose, I cannot bend too much, and if it is too tight, I do not feel at ease and it shows that one side is flatter than the other. It has become a daily chore to choose an appropriate outfit.

It has been a year now since the verdict has been given. When I think back on what I have been going through, it almost seems unreal to me.

There were some difficult steps, like losing my hair, but also some positive sides to the disease.

I have met amazing people, embraced a new way of looking at things, and learnt how to deal with stress better.

A year later, I meet a young lady suffering from the same disease, who will have to overcome the same obstacles I went through. I know she will make it, and I hope that she will be as determined as I was.

The earlier the cancer is spotted, the lighter and lesser the consequences. But as long as we do not feel threatened, we do not think about any of this. We do not think about either the risks, or the consequences.

CHAPTER 17. CHECK-UP WITH THE RADIOTHERAPIST

The month of March would be synonymous with stress, anxiety and tears.
It all started with some bleeding after ten months without being on my period. The radiotherapist had warned me that it could happen because of the hormone therapy. She had also told me that should it happen, I would have to do a pelvic ultrasound scan. The medicstion could indeed trigger a cancer of the uterus. As the probability of such a thing to happen is much lower than the breast cancer coming back, I had made up my mind quickly.

The ultrasound scan carried out some days later displays a thickened endometrium with a few cysts on the edge.

I hence meet with the gynaecologist at the cancer centre where I am taken care of. She reassures me and explains that this situation happens quite often. To be sure, she prescribes a cleaning-out of the endometrium. I should undergo the surgery under general anaesthesia but, with her authorisation, I ask to try to undergo it under hypnosis, to avoid sedation.

Even if I try to stay upbeat, I keep in mind the fact that everything could collapse again.

Since I have started to get the injections of Herceptin, heart scans are scheduled every three months. They usually all look the same, but this time, on the 11th of March, it is different. I tell the cardiologist about my symptoms, and about the fact that I stopped doing the injections at home. He places the captors on my body, carries out the examination and does not say a word. He removes all the captors and then puts them back. While his machine is on, he asks me if I feel good and if I get easily out of breath. It is true that it has happened to me at times, but I am not really into sports, so it had seemed normal. But was it really?

"Strange," he says while starring at the results. I can feel my heart beating faster and faster, and a knot forming in my stomach.

He carries on with the heart scan, which will thankfully turn out to be normal.

The cardiologist explains to me that on the scan, there is no relevant modification, a fact that is reassuring. But as the ECG showed a modification, I will have to do a heart MRI anyway, to make sure that my heart can handle the treatment.

After having received the results, the oncologist decides to suspend the injections, in agreement with his colleagues. To resume the treatment, I will have to wait for the MRI. It puts me in a very stressful and uncomfortable position. I have been told since the beginning that this treatment was key, so having to stop it for a while worries me a lot.

I am overwhelmed and start crying. I am bad-tempered, angry and stressed out for a few days. It is too much in too short a period. The time I have to wait before the MRI does not make things better. When I first try to make an appointment, I am told that it would not be possible to do so before the end of July. But I insist, explain my situation thoroughly and eventually succeed in making an appointment for the end of May. My despair about the situation even pushes the doctors to give me an appointment on the 29th of March. I am told the same day that my heart MRI is normal.

The oncologist then calls me to tell me that I will be able to resume the injections. I have five left to do. It is one thing less that I have to think about, and I feel much lighter.

On the 9th of May 2019, six months after the end of radiotherapy, I meet again with the specialist. I explain to him everything that has happened recently: the break in my injections of Herceptin, the heart MRI... I also tell him about the intervention scheduled fifteen days from now, to sample my endometrium.

He is very reassuring:

"I am not worried at all. You would need to take the tablets several years to face a serious risk to get cancer."

"You are cheering me up Doctor, but the gynaecologist wants to be a hundred per cent sure about it."

"Of course, and you will have to get your endometrium sampled, but you should not worry about it."

He adds:

"However, you are supposed to meet with the surgeon in June, and it is way too early. Actually, you should be seeing the specialists alternately every three months: the surgeon, the oncologist and myself. I will postpone the appointment with the surgeon to November."

"I was thinking it was strange to see everyone in two months as well."

"Yes, and we are going to change this. We will do the same for the first mammography scheduled in June. I will postpone it to November as well."

"No, I would like to stick with the appointment for the mammography. It has been scheduled at this date for a while and I have been preparing for it. I need to be reassured thanks to this check-up, as it will be the first since the beginning of the disease. I have been waiting for it for a while."

"As you wish, you can stick with it if you like."

I do not get flustered. I would not have dared speaking up before, but right now, I have the feeling that it is too important to stay quiet. I cannot even think about postponing it, as I need to hear that the cancer is gone and that it will not come back.

He continues:

"How is the hormone therapy going?"

"I'm doing fine. I sometimes get tired a bit quicker than I used to, but could it be due to the injections of Herceptin?"

"Indeed, the treatments you have been undergoing are very heavy, and your body might take at least a year to purge them out."

"I'm not surprised."

"Perfect, we will see each other again in a year from now."

"Thank you Doctor, see you next year!"

CHAPTER 18. SAMPLING THE ENDOMETRIUM

The 15th of May, the day I will get my endometrium sampled, is fast approaching.

Today it's Monday the 13th, I have a missed call from the hospital and a voice message on my answering machine:

"Good morning, I am calling you on the behalf of the surgery department, to move your arrival time from 7.30 a.m. to 7.15 a.m. The surgery has been scheduled for 8 a.m. Thank you and have a good day."

I'm a bit stressed out. But in the end, it might be better to undergo the surgery as soon as I arrive, so that I will not have much time to think about it.

I get up at 5.30 a.m. and take a shower while listening to music. I am calm, relaxed, and quite surprised about being so!

At 6.15 a.m., the shuttle comes. We chit chat on the way to the hospital.

At 7.15 a.m., I am at the hospital. I get set up in a room and am also shown the safe to put my personal belongings in. Thefts are apparently common, a fact

I cannot wrap my head around. How can you possibly imagine being stolen from at the hospital, while you are on the operating table? Crazy.

I put on the outfit I know so well now. Blue scrubs, as well as a blue paper robe. The porter comes to pick me up and accompanies me to the waiting room next to the operating block.

A nurse takes charge of me and brings me to the block itself. Both the anaesthetist and the nurses are getting busy around me in order to get me ready for the upcoming surgery. One of the nurses then explains to me that I will be under an anaesthetic. My heart skips a beat and I say with a shaking voice:

"No! I was supposed to undergo the surgery under hypnosis."

"I am sorry Madam, but we will have to proceed under general anaesthesia. Nothing is specified in your file regarding hypnosis, and the people who are skilled in the field are absent today."

"I understand. I guess I will have to sleep then," I answer with a laugh.

I understand quickly where the mistake comes from. When I rescheduled the appointment with the surgeon, after having gone through the heart MRI, she did not think about hypnosis and neither did I. I did not think about reminding her about it either during the days that followed the MRI.

I have mixed feelings about the situation. I am upset about the change of plan, but at the same time,

I was afraid that the hypnosis would not work. I have to come to terms with it anyway, I do not have the choice.

An oxygen mask is placed on my mouth, I feel calm. I take a deep breath. I get the injection and my head starts spinning. I panic, It feels like I am sinking into the bed. Everything becomes blurry. I hate this feeling of not being in control, of having to let go and rely entirely on the medical staff.

"Madam! Madam! Time to wake up!"
I try to open my eyes, but they weigh a ton. I try to answer but I am still feeling too weak to do so.
The nurse's voice echoes in my head:

"You are in the recovery room and everything went as planned. You can wake up peacefully and you will soon be brought back to your room."

"Thanks," I whisper.

A porter brings me back to my room. I try to surface several times, but I keep on falling back asleep.

At noon, a nurse comes and tells me that I would be able to leave by 2 p.m. She brings me some breakfast: bread with butter, some coffee and an apple juice. I eat a bit before taking another nap.

At 1.30 p.m., the intern in surgery comes to sign my authorisation to leave, and tells me softly with a big smile on his face:

"The surgeon asked me to tell you that everything went well, and that everything seems normal inside." The samples will give us a more accurate answer, but she seems optimistic.

"Alright, thank you very much," I answer, reassured and a bit more confident.

At 3.30 p.m., I am back home, delighted to be with my husband.

Tonight, I will sleep at my parents' place with my children, as my husband is working night shifts and the hospital does not want me to spend the first night alone.

I slept well, even if my night was quite agitated. At least, the pain is bearable.

The following days, I rest and nap a lot.

One morning, after having used my left arm a bit too much, it swells and becomes painful. The lymph does not flow properly, due to the ganglion cleanout that was carried out at the same time as the mastectomy. My doctor prescribes physiotherapy sessions twice a week and I have to wear a cuff. A cuff looks like a support stocking, but it is built for the upper limbs. You can easily imagine how hard it is to put it on every morning. After some days though, I get used to it. It is part of me and soothes my pain quite well.

According to the physiotherapist, I will have to wait for the end of the summer to get rid of it, as the heat causes the limbs to swell even more.

CHAPTER 19. THE LONG-AWAITED RESULTS

Tomorrow, the verdict will be given. I have been waiting for my DNA results for a year now. My stress level increases, because if I do carry a gene, it would bring about various consequences.

Among other things, I could have transmitted it to my daughter, and I also could have to remove both my other breast and my uterus. I am already imagining what would be my reaction if it was the case. To realise that you could have passed on something so negative and dangerous to your own child is not easy. As usual, I try to think positive.

The big plus about getting tested and knowing whether you carry the gene or not, is to be taken in charge earlier and better, as well as to be able to monitor your children's health better when they grow up. In the end, the earlier it is detected, the better.

I am calm but thoughtful on my way to the appointment. The two possibilities get tangled in my head. I am still thinking about it when the doctor shows up and tells me to come into her office. She starts by explaining again what the three types of genes they have looked for are. I am listening to her but cannot help thinking that it is probably not a good sign if she is taking time to do so.

I feel relieved when she eventually tells me:

"The good news is that the test came back negative. And it is ninety-eight to ninety-nine percent reliable."

More than relieved, I am overjoyed... for my daughter and for myself.

She adds that I could ask to run another test that would look for a fourth gene. The latter can affect children, boys or girls, and trigger tumours. She gives me lots of information and tells me that I can think about it before agreeing to proceed with the test. They think that my risk rate would be around ten percent. I answer:

"I understood what you have told me, and I want to do the test. If it turns out to be positive, my children could be affected. If I do not do it and find out in the future that they have something, I would blame myself for the rest of my life. So I agree, there is nothing more to think about."

Since the beginning of the sickness, it has been the same. One appointment has always led to another, as well as to new expectations, new questions. It gives you the feeling that it will never stop.

I went to the appointment thinking that, if I was not carrying any of those three genes, I was going to be relieved. But in the end, I have to wait for yet another result.

Six months is a long time when you are waiting for something, so I will try not to think about it too much, and to enjoy every single moment of happiness. And they are numerous.

When everything is going fine in our life, we do not think about the daily little joys, but we should.

Some birds' songs, the beauty of nature, an enjoyable conversation, drinking coffee while sitting in the sun, reading a good book... These things become so important once you have thought that you might not be able to do any of them again. Life is so beautiful, live it to the fullest!

Six days later, the result of the endometrium sampling is waiting for me. Since the day of the surgery, I have been feeling reassured. The gynaecologist had not seen anything abnormal, so I was calm, or almost so.

But today is different. Nothing had foretold my breast cancer, so it could be the same right now.

I've had a knot in my stomach from the moment I woke up. I am scared of having to go through all this again.

When I arrive, the secretary tells me that they are behind schedule. The wait is endless, and even if I am trying to keep my mind busy, I can feel my stress slowly taking over.

An hour and a half later, it is finally my turn. I know that doctors have to deal with emergencies and can be late, but I am fuming. Waiting that long while asking myself so many questions is unbearable.

She invites me in and asks me how I feel. I answer that I am feeling alright, despite the increased stress level due to the waiting time. She understands and apologises.

However, I calm down quickly when she tells me that my results came back normal. What a relief!

My stress comes down immediately, and both my smile and my good mood come back in an instant.

A series of good news that rejoices me. Long may it last!

CHAPTER 20. A FORTUNATE ENCOUNTER

It's now the 12th of May, and I must tell you how fantastic my taxi ride back home was.

I am just done with my injection of Herceptin, and my head's in the clouds but I am still feeling alright for the moment.

The taxi is here, it is waiting for me and two women are waiting as well. We are all going back together, as our houses are located in the same direction.

I sit at the back of the vehicle. One of the two women sits at the front, and the other one on my right-hand side. The latter is moving with difficulty and uses a walking stick. She tells me that she has been having health problems for a while now, and that she previously had to spend several years in a wheelchair. She is easy-going. I identify with her, as learning that I was sick freed me in a way. I now feel free to do what I want, when and where I want it, without caring about what people think, provided that it brings me joy and satisfaction.

She is fond of Johnny Halliday, and I understand it as soon as I hear the song *Marie*, playing on the radio. She starts singing immediately, as if she was on her own. Nothing seems to be disturbing her. It only takes me a few seconds to start singing along.

I really cannot sing, but I do not care at all and am just enjoying myself. How wonderful it is to feel content!

We do not know each other, but we are sharing an amazing moment thanks to the music. We keep on singing for the rest of the thirty-minute journey.

I will never forget it. It was such a wonderful moment.

The month of June has just started, and the weather is amazing today, so I take advantage of it to pick up my children from school by foot. While on my way, I meet a woman walking her dog, her daughter is in a stroller. While our respective dogs are getting acquainted, the woman calls out to me:

"Do we know each other?"

"Indeed! We were in the same class in high school!"

"What's up with you?"

I go blank. I feel as if I was taking a jump in the blue. What should I answer when my life has been revolving around my disease for the past year? The silence goes thicker when I eventually mutter:

"What's up with me? Well, I am a playschool assistant and am currently on a long sick leave."

"Alright. You have changed your haircut. It changes you a lot. How are you?"

I am quite embarrassed and answer:

"I am doing well thank you. What about you?"

"I am good. Let me introduce you to my nine-month-old daughter."

"She is adorable! Congratulations then!"

"Thanks. Are you having health issues?"

"I had breast cancer about a year and a half ago but I am feeling much better now."

It is her turn to go blank and to feel awkward.

We have not seen each other for fifteen years, so we keep on chatting. She seems to have problems as well. She tells me that she is having a hard time controlling her level of stress, and that it is driving her crazy.

I know exactly where she is coming from. I know the feeling all too well from having experienced the same.

I tell her that I used to be exactly like her, but that since I have been sick, stress has been replaced with freedom and a relaxed attitude.

On these words of wisdom, I have to go pick up my children, but we decide to stay in touch and to see each other again.

On my way, I think back on the discussion, and cannot help but think that our meeting was not just a random one. In a whole year, we met only once, despite the fact that our town is fairly small and that we live five hundred metres away from each other.

Isn't it strange? Is it a sign? Maybe I could help her to feel better? Feeling understood by someone who went through the same troubles can help sometimes.

"There is always be a reason why you meet people. Either you need them to change your life, or you are the one they need to change theirs." The quote is from Angel Flonis Harefa.

Anyway, I am delighted with this unexpected meeting.

CHAPTER 21. MY REFLECTION IN THE MIRROR

It is the 14th of June and I meet with the cardiologist for the first time since my heart MRI. I wait apprehensively in the waiting room. Then, the specialist makes me go into his office and starts carrying out the electrocardiogram, the latter turning out to be normal this time. According to him, the reason why it was not last time was because the Herceptin had caused an arrythmia. Stopping the product for a while considerably improved my physical and psychological health, I could not have coped with it much longer.

The heart scan comes next. I have to wait for a while before the specialist reassures me, telling me that everything is normal as well.

I have only one injection of Herceptin left on the 2nd of July, before being able to enjoy my freedom fully. The end of all the treatments, except for the hormone therapy, will be pure pleasure. The three last injections have gone just fine. I still feel very tired during one or two days but recover much quicker.

I come back from the appointment serene, happy and feeling brave. I feel young and in shape. One thing is sure, heart and life go hand in hand, and knowing that my heart is healthy brings back my strength and vitality.

It has been almost two months since I've been having appointments twice a week with the physiotherapist to work on my lymphoedema, as well as on my chest and shoulder. With the surgery, the scar and the lack of physical effort on this side, my muscles got stiff. The sessions last an hour, they are long, straining and time-consuming, but also crucial for the breast reconstruction to come.

Today, she gives me an exercise to relax my neck and shoulder, which have been hurting for a few days now. She puts a chair in front of a big mirror and asks me to take off my top. So far so good, I am used to it. I sit on the chair and see my reflection in the mirror. It strikes me hard when I notice that I have put on a paunch and two love handles. I am not even mentioning my thighs, as I barely recognise them.

It is seeing my entire body which is strange, as I usually only see myself in the mirror down to the shoulders. During the session, I stare at my reflection and try to stand tall… but it is of no use. It is not that surprising, I have been putting on weight because of the hormone therapy, but I had not realised how much.

With the return of a warmer weather and the end of the injections, I will focus on walking and taking strolls during the summer. My new goal: lose some weight.

During the following days, I find more energy as well as a greater stamina. The reassuring diagnosis of the cardiologist and the realisation of how my body looked motivate me, and I take walks more regularly.

CHAPTER 22. FIRST GENERAL CHECK-UP

In four days, I will undergo the first general check-up since I have learnt about my disease. It is going to be my first mammography in a year and a half, the first since my life has been turned upside-down. I cannot wait, I want to know that there is nothing vicious left inside my body, nothing more to fight, and that I can lay down my weapons. The specialists feel my breast at each appointment, as I know all too well, it is possible to have something without it being noticed.

A nightmare ruined my night. It seemed so real that I believed it was true. I woke up with a knot in my stomach and a heart rate going through the roof. I dreamt that the mammography was not good and that I was having a relapse. It was disturbing and stressful. I tried to forget about it when I woke up, but it was too late. And now I cannot calm down.

Today is the the 26th of June. It is 3.30 p.m., and a technician guides me to the room where the mammography will be carried out. I am quite confident, but she comes back ten minutes later and tells me:

"Your breast is too dense, we will have to do an ultrasound scan."

The pressure goes up, it is hard to breathe and the heat is not helping. I follow her, enter another room, and the radiologist carries out the scan. She is the same person who told me, a year and a half ago, that I had another tumour. I have a flash back. I feel exactly the same, I am as stressed out as I was back then. She tells me:

"Everything is normal, your next mammography will be scheduled in a year. You will have to go through an ultrasound scan as well."

I am overjoyed. Yes, I can lay down my weapons, while keeping them in sight, just in case. I understand that I can have a relapse, but I am enjoying the present moment, and above all, I am enjoying life.

I meet with the oncologist and an hour and a half later, she backs up the first result. She also reminds me that I have one injection of Herceptin left and that I should go through a heart check-up every six months. However, given what happened to me, she prefers seeing me in four months and do the heart check-up right after.

I send a message to my parents and to my husband immediately, as they have also been anxiously waiting for the result.

The ride back home was very enjoyable, with a friendly ambulance driver who had a great sense of humour. I keep both my smile and my good mood all night long. Coming back home, I give my husband a hug, full of satisfaction and happiness. Then, I explain to my children:

"I did a check-up with the doctor and everything is normal. Your mummy is not sick anymore."
My daughter reacts:

"So you are not carrying any more germs?"

"They were not germs, but you are right though, I have nothing nasty left in my body."

"And if it comes back, you will go through chemotherapy again?"
Her comment shows that children understand a lot. I had never told her about a possible relapse, but my seven-year-old daughter understood perfectly that it could happen.

"You are right my love. But I am doing everything I can for it not to come back. It is also why I am taking tablets every night."

The next check-up is next year, but waiting for it, I intend to enjoy my life fully.

CHAPTER 23. SOME WORDS TO CONCLUDE

I wanted to cancel my gynaecological appointment a few days before it was supposed to take place, and it would have been a mistake. I had to make the appointment so far ahead that when the actual date of the appointment came, I got lazy and did not want to go, especially because my husband was on holidays. But he told me to go and insisted on it. It is a blessing that he did so, otherwise things would have been pretty different for me.

That is why I consider myself lucky to have discovered that I had cancer early enough. Even though the treatments would have been lighter if I had found out even earlier. Now, I always try to look at the bright side of any situation. And there always is one…

The disease showed me whom I could trust and unfortunately, I apparently cannot trust the two people I considered to be my best friends. They were not there for me, and there is now a distance between us. They sent me messages such as 'Hello, what's up?' I did not think that this type of message was appropriate.

When I lost my hair, I could rely only on myself and my family. As they did not reach out to me, I could not see myself writing to them to look for comfort during such a difficult period. Consequently, they learnt about it only a few months later. They also hinted that it would be too difficult for them to see me like this. But I am not the one to blame, they should have been even more present in my life.

I do not know if they did it on purpose or if they just did not know how to react, but the result is the same. I cannot see the point of keeping them by my side, as I only want to be around positive and supportive people now.

On the contrary, acquaintances, former work colleagues, parents from my children's school, shared their compassion and support in multiple ways and helped me stay strong.

My family, unsurprisingly, was really there for me. And it is what matters the most to me. As the saying goes, 'You can choose your friends, but you do not choose your family'. I can still make new friends, on whom I will be able to lean this time.

My husband and my children were a real driving force. They pushed me to go forward.

From my husband's viewpoint, it has probably been terrible to see me changing like this. My body was maimed, and a big scar replaced a nice-looking breast. I do not even want to talk about my hair. I went from having long, dark blond hair to being bald. Then, my hair grew again but black and curly. Then, the hormone therapy made me put on weight, and I grew two graceless love handles. But I am not giving up, I am going to get the grip back on my life, as I am alive and healthy now. And that is the most important thing.

My husband kept on looking at me with love and desire despite all the physical changes I went through, and I am so grateful for it. Our love came out stronger.

Not disappointing my family and healing had become my two main goals lately.

Now I live my life imagining a happiness gauge that I would fill up with various daily pleasures. And as I said earlier, there are so many of them…every day. We just tend to forget about them because we are caught in a routine and are not paying attention to what is around us. We are always running after time, whether it is for work, to pick-up our children at school or to do the housework. Most lives are orchestrated by an accumulation of daily micro-tasks that prevent people from focusing on what really matters, and from enjoying all the great things that life has to offer.

As far as I am concerned, the tiniest pleasure can fill up my happiness gauge: a bird landing in my garden, a little snail popping its head out and making its way on the ledge of my window, a hug from my children, an enjoyable conversation, a good meal in a nice restaurant… I have learnt how to be filled with wonder at the simplest things, and how to enjoy my days fully. We never know what tomorrow will bring, and one's life can stop in the blink of an eye. I have become aware of it.

Now it is your turn…